Beatiful Skin

Everything you need to know about skin care and nobody has explained it to you

Beautiful Skin

Table Of Contents

Chapter 1

Introduction

Let's face the fact: Many of us are skin conscious. As much as possible, we want to have fresh and attractive skin. However, many of us cannot recognize that simple steps are the best ways to achieve this. We just tend to ignore what is really right or wrong for our skin. We tend to buy some beauty products that worsen the skin blemishes that we have at the end. So now is the time for change. We must do something to beat all those pesky skin conditions we have.

Think and act CLEAN

One thing that is certain in our society from the earliest days is that some, if not all, companies that produce skin care products would like you to believe that you can buy a perfect and beautiful complexion in a jar. But the truth is that truly radiant, blemish-free and moist skin is the result of being clean. If I say "clean", it means clean from the deep and not just on the skin.

Most medical professionals commonly suggest that people with skin problems should practice certain skin care methods that will help improve the skin condition. One of the most recommended ways is to gently cleanse the skin by washing it with a mild cleanser, at least once in the morning and once at night, as well as after intense training. But behind that, there is one thing that is crucial to maintaining beautiful skin, and that is: creating clean blood that continuously supplies wonderful nutrients directly to the door of each and every cell in your body. If you will start practicing this, there is no doubt that you are on your way to beautiful skin.

But how can you make it possible?

Well, these days, keeping toxins out of the blood and body organs seems difficult. The main reason is that most of us live in a "sea" of chemicals and drugs. We even mainly eat refined foods. Now if your primary "target" is healthy, beautiful skin, then it's time for you to make a conscious effort to flush these dangerous substances out of your system while putting in the best nutrients. There is one particular good news that you should know about your own system, meaning your body is constantly in a cleaning mode. It was created with the ability to expel toxins as long as the necessary energy is supplied to make it work.

The bottom line is: cleansing energy is most abundant when you supply your body with nutritious food. Note the word "nutritious".

Main organs that keep your skin beautiful

Our body is made up of different organs responsible for providing us with beautiful and healthy skin. These specifically include:

- Liver
- Kidneys
- Kidney glands
- Thyroid
- Large intestines
- Small intestines

Please note that with these mentioned organs, you are also responsible to them. It is now your role to keep them clean at all times. In the end you will discover that beautiful skin will result from your daily efforts.

Liver and kidneys

It is interesting to know that our liver and kidneys are the two filtering organs that constantly provide "house cleaning services", as I prefer to constantly call it. You should be aware that these days these organs are very worn out and even underpaid. So why overload them with external challenges? Do you find it difficult to protect them from external damage? However, it is not that difficult. Just feed them well and they'll keep it, including their healthy skin at the end.

Kidney glands

Also, above your kidneys are your walnut-sized adrenal glands. These organs are often called the "workhorses" of the human body, perhaps for the reason that they are responsible for producing a number of essential hormones such as DHEA, estrogen, progesterone, testosterone, and pregnenolone. Speaking of hormones, it is necessary to keep in mind that healthy hormones are the essential ingredient when looking for energy, as well as healthy skin.

Thyroid

It is often said that if your thyroid is well-nourished and energetic, it is capable of providing hormones and works closely with your adrenal glands to form essential energy. Keep in mind that dry, slow, flaky skin is actually evidence of a weak thyroid. Therefore, strengthen it.

Large and small intestines

Studies have revealed that the general well-being of the liver, kidneys, adrenal glands, and thyroid depends on the general condition of the small and large intestine. In addition to supplying nutrients to these organs, the small and large intestines have a responsibility to eliminate any accumulated waste products in the body. If the small and large intestines do not fulfill this function, the waste destined for elimination will remain in your intestines and this will cause a thickening of the skin, which will eventually produce oils and blemishes. Clean intestines actually reflect pure, flawless skin.

Various reports have pointed out that drugs, alcohol, chemicals, and heavy metals like mercury and lead cause daily harm to millions of people around the world. The liver is mainly damaged by refined oils that contain trans fatty acids, while the kidneys are damaged by common table salt that lacks natural minerals. Perhaps the main reason for this is the fact that thousands of processed foods that people often consume every day have trans fat and refined salt. Additionally, it was found that pasteurized and homogenized dairy products tend to clog the kidneys, so they should be avoided. But, to achieve healthy and beautiful skin, you should definitely add foods to your diet that nourish the above six organs of beauty.

Think green

Today, there is what many dermatologists call "Spring". In Chinese medicine, spring is the season when the liver is naturally cleansed and healed by expelling dangerous toxins that accumulate in the body through the refined foods we eat. Many experts suggest green foods, including Chlorella, as they are said to be excellent for the liver. Keep in mind that green foods refer to green leafy vegetables like spinach, kale, dandelion, and broccoli. These foods are what many people consider "especially wonderful foods." Now for healthy and beautiful skin, make them cooked, raw, squeezed, and even cultivated.

More food needed to nourish your body and skin

In general, superfood formulas provide a mix of nutrients necessary for the body and skin. These include cereal grasses, algae, and green vegetables. Therefore, it is best that you look for one that contains organic ingredients, but also keep in mind that the food was designed to heal and nourish the small and large intestines. Such foods are often said to be ideal in the morning because they help the blood become alkaline. Also, they are nice to take a handful of supplements. They even provide minerals, fatty acids, and protein to the body.

Other foods known to contribute to healthy skin include raw and virgin fats and oils. A perfect source in particular is coconut oil, which is especially good for the thyroid. Also, mineral-rich foods like dark green leafy vegetables, ocean vegetables, and seafood are important. And, antioxidant-rich foods like blackcurrant and cranberry juice and green tea are also a daily necessity.

Also, there is one more group of foods worth mentioning: fermented or cultured foods. In reality, these foods are found in all traditional cultures around the world and many have considered them the protagonists of a healthy diet. Like some of the foods mentioned above, they are necessary to maintain healthy and wonderful skin.

Chapter 2

What is natural skin care?

Simply put, 'natural skin care' is taking care of your skin in a natural and chemical-free way. 'Natural skin care' advocates allowing the skin to take care of itself (without the help of synthetic / chemical materials). 'Natural skin care' consists of instilling good habits in the way you carry out your daily life. Many natural measures for skin care are actually the same as for general body care.

So let's see what these natural measures for skin care are.

The first and most important natural measure for skin care is: "Drink plenty of water." About 8 glasses of water are a must every day. Water helps flush toxins from the body naturally. It helps in the general maintenance of the body and promotes the good health of all the organs (not only the skin).

General cleaning is another inexpensive form of natural skin care. Daily showering, wearing clean clothes and sleeping on a clean mattress / pillow are part of the general cleaning. After all, clean skin is the key to keeping skin disorders at bay.

Regular exercise is next on the cards. Exercise increases blood flow that helps flush toxins from the body and keep it healthy. Exercise also helps fight stress, which is the worst enemy of good health.

Healthy foods and eating habits are also recommended for natural skin care. Some type of food (eg, fatty foods) is known to cause acne and should be avoided as much as possible. Your diet should be a healthy mix of various nutrients-providing foods. Raw fruits and vegetables are known to provide freshness to your body and help flush toxins out of the body.

Good sleep is also essential to maintain good health and combat stress. As a natural skin care measure, good sleep delays skin looseness.

Overcoming stress is another natural skin care therapy. Stress causes general damage to the body and health. Drinking plenty of water, sleeping well, and exercising has already been mentioned as a stressor. Enjoying a warm bubble bath, listening to music and practicing your favorite sport are also good ways to combat stress. Yoga is another way to overcome stress; it is rapidly gaining popularity among the masses.

Avoiding excessive sun exposure (wearing long-sleeved clothing, a hat and an umbrella, etc.) is another natural skin care strategy. Sunscreen lotions are also recommended as needed.

Many traditional and natural skin care products / measures are also known to be very effective. Such measures are not only natural and easy to follow, but are also relatively inexpensive.

In addition to that, many natural skin care products are available in the commercial market. These include things like lavender oil, aloe vera, etc., that don't have any side effects.

Chapter 3

Transforming into the natural

The benefits of jojoba oil

When making the decision to switch to a more natural skincare routine, you may be surprised to learn about all the benefits of jojoba oil.

For starters, it is not comedogenic. Which means it won't clog your pores.

This is especially good news for those of us with sensitive skin, the kind that tends to break easily without the use of facial oil.

And part of your skincare routine is to remove excess dirt and oil from your face, so knowing that a natural oil won't cause buildup is a huge plus.

Other benefits of jojoba oil is that structurally speaking, it is incredibly similar to the natural sebum your own skin produces.

That is why so many people use it as a daily moisturizer, seeing how it comes directly from nature.

If you're someone who often wears makeup, then here is yet another reason to add jojoba oil to your skincare, it's a game changer when it comes to removing stubborn makeup.

This means that instead of using makeup remover wipes even before you wash your face, a quick application of jojoba oil will do the trick.

And this is also good for the environment, as you add those wipes to your trash or septic system.

If those two benefits haven't convinced you to incorporate jojoba oil into your natural skincare routine, then maybe it's will.

Jojoba oil is packed with natural anti-inflammatory properties.

Skin inflammation occurs when you've also been out in the sun a long time, perhaps with little or no sunscreen, and your skin burns in the sun. Aloe vera will help, but so will jojoba oil.

Or maybe you have been itching a pimple or you have a wound on your face that has become irritated. Try applying a little jojoba oil to see if the natural anti-inflammatory and properties help calm the skin.

You can easily find jojoba oil in whole food stores, health stores, and even beauty retailers. Look for ones that are 100% natural and try it on a small part of your skin first.

The benefits of oats

If you've ever taken a look at all of the bath and body products in your pharmacy, then you've probably seen a lot that contain oatmeal.

That is because it is considered to be of an exfoliating nature. But before you go rubbing some of the quick cook oatmeal you probably have in your pantry all over your body, you should know that they are different from what we are talking about Colloidal Oatmeal.

The Administration (FDA) approves as a natural way to treat dry skin. Especially if you have eczema, which is an extreme form of medically diagnosed dry skin.

So if your skin needs a little hydration, read on to learn about ways to use colloidal oatmeal as part of your natural skincare routine.

If you decide to use freshly ground, colloidal oatmeal, and then here is an idea to use it as a full body scrub.

Simply mix a little with local organic honey, add a little water, and then apply it to your clean skin, focusing on extremely dry areas like your elbows and knees. Massage for about a minute, and then rinse with warm water and pat dry.

You can also use it on your face. Apply the same mixture to your freshly cleaned skin, massaging for about a minute and then rinse.

If the soles of your feet, especially the soles of your feet, often get dry, then this is a great way to smooth them up. Just use the same mixture while doing a foot bath.

You can also prepare a little in advance and put it in a jar, then leave it on your skin. Just use it as a hand scrub every time you wash.

Soap and water can actually dry out your skin, so use it as often as possible.

Of course, there are also many skincare brands.

They use colloidal oatmeal as one of their main ingredients.

These are just a few ways to use all-natural oatmeal colloids as part of your skincare routine.

The benefits of raw honey

We constantly hear about the many benefits of raw, unprocessed honey. But it turns out that it is also very good for your skin.

There are many antibacterial products on the market, and sometimes you need that kind of treatment for your face. But instead of applying something that is commercially done with added chemicals, try this next time.

Thoroughly clean the stain on your skin that needs antibacterial treatment, then apply a teaspoon of raw honey to the area and gently massage into the skin. Let it sit for 10 minutes and then rinse with warm water Repeat until the infection is gone.

The same type of treatment can be used as a mask as well.

After removing all makeup, take a teaspoon of honey and gently work on your face. And don't worry about your skin getting naked. Honey is very relaxing, so it won't hurt your face at all. Let it sit for 10 minutes and then rinse it off with lukewarm water, just like a regular mask

Raw honey is also anti-inflammatory. Sometimes our skin needs a little cooling, and when you are looking to adopt a more natural way to the skin care routine you want, avoid chemicals

So if an area of your body is irritated and inflamed, just take a teaspoon of honey and let it sit for 10 minutes or so, just like other treatments, and then rinse it off with lukewarm water.

Whenever possible, try to buy locally sourced honey. Just make sure it's raw and unprocessed.

If you really feel luxurious, then consider using raw honey as a mask on other parts of your body as well. Like your legs, arms, and even your neck. It's not just our face that needs some love!

If you still want to buy products in a pharmacy, be sure to look for those that contain raw honey. There are many brands out there that use this delicious nectar in their products.

These are just a few ways to use all natural, raw honey as part of your skincare routine.

The benefits of papaya

As we age, we tend to develop more skin problems, such as sun spots and large pores. And if you are looking for a more natural skincare routine, these could be concerns that need to be addressed.

The good news is that papaya cares for multiple skin needs.

This delicious bright orange fruit is packed with many benefits.

By applying papaya as a mask on your face, it actually helps to equalize your skin tone. Just think about the good, your skin will look without makeup after a few papaya masks the same goes for your pores.

While it's important to spray and clean, get your pores out every now and then, no one wants them to be big. That is why we use products on our face to minimize the appearance of our pores.

But a papaya mask can actually help shrink your pores, which means you can. You don't have to wear as much makeup!

If you are over 40, then you may very well have some sun spots on your skin too.

It is only part of aging and yes, the foundation can cover it. But a papaya mask can actually get to the source of the problem and get rid of them over time.

To try this amazing and natural skincare form, simply mash about 1/4 of a ripe banana with a tablespoon of raw, all-natural organic honey and let it sit in the refrigerator for about an hour.

Then apply it on your clean face, relax and let it sit for about 20 minutes and then rinse it off with lukewarm water.

To get the most out of this papaya mask, try doing this once or twice a week and notice the difference over time.

Papayas are also quite large fruits, so you can get more than one treatment for each.

These are just a few ways to use delicious papayas as part of your natural skincare routine.

The benefits of cucumber

There's a reason you constantly see people in spa ads with cucumber slices under their eyes, smiling as they relax with a large towel.

This vegetable is really a gift from Mother Nature to our bodies.

In addition to being good for your physique and health when consumed, cucumbers are saturated with antioxidants that can do wonders for your skin when applied topically.

I have mentioned that antioxidants are perfect for reducing skin irritation. This is why you should add cucumbers to your natural skincare routine.

Just take a few slices of cold cucumber and place them on the part of your skin that is irritated for about 5-10 minutes. It can take some applications. And of course please consult your doctor for any long-term skin irritation.

If you are one of the millions of people in this world suffering from allergies, then you should absolutely add cucumbers to your natural skincare as a routine!

With seasonal allergies, puffy eyes often appear and all you need to do is apply a slice of cucumber to each of your eyelids and wait about 5-10 minutes. And you should also keep your eyes closed.

Then remove the slices and massage any cucumber juice into your skin. Not only will your eyes look more refreshed, but you will be amazed at how much better they feel!

Another great benefit of cucumbers is that they are loaded with water, which is perfect for reducing bloating.

Some people suffer from swollen ankles, and while water and elevating the feet will often help, it is also a good idea to apply some sliced cold cucumber to them as well.

Keep them elevated and wait about 5-10 minutes, just like the other home remedies, and then massage any cucumber juice into your ankles.

This is especially good if you are a woman who suffers from water retention during her menstrual cycle. Consider doing it more often during those times of the month, if necessary.

These are just a few ways to use refreshing cucumbers as part of your natural skincare routine.

The benefits of turmeric

So far we have discussed the natural healing and benefits of fruits and vegetables for your skin.

And now is the time to spice things up.

Literally!

Turmeric is a bright orange spice that is often used to flavor foods, but its natural anti-inflammatory properties can also do wonders for your skin.

For example, those suffering from acne should consider using turmeric as a face mask.

Not only can it help lighten the breakouts you have, but it has been shown to reduce scarring as well.

The same properties that tackle acne can also reduce the size of your pores!

Not only are the smaller pores a bit more attractive than the larger ones, but they also won't be able to retain as much dirt and oil. Which is equivalent to scrubbing your face less, which is always a good thing because it pulls on your skin!

And just like other natural products I've talked about, turmeric can also soothe your skin.

For mild skin irritation, try applying a little turmeric powder mixed with warm water and applying it for about 10 minutes or so, then rinse off.

If you have any of these skincare problems, or even if you only have oily skin that needs help, try mixing turmeric with rose water and applying as a mask.

Of course, thoroughly clean the area before using the mask and be sure to rinse it well. Any long-term skin problem should always be addressed by a healthcare provider.

Over time, the more you use turmeric powder as part of your natural skincare routine, the more you will see the benefits.

And to make sure it doesn't irritate your skin, try a small patch of skin with a little turmeric powder and warm water. If it doesn't get itchy or burning, slowly start using it as a mask.

These are just a few ways to use healing turmeric as part of your natural skincare routine.

The benefits of pineapple juice

We will discuss why integrating pineapple juice, as uncomfortable

As it may sound, it could give your face a glow.

First of all, it is important to know that pineapple juice is quite acidic. Please test it on a small portion of your skin or meet with a healthcare provider first.

One of the best things about pineapple juice, other than tasting so good, is that it is anti-aging. And you really should start your anti-aging treatment as early as twenty years old.

If you haven't already and you are new, there is no need to worry.

Try some pineapple juice on a cotton ball and gently place it on your clean face. Bromelain, Vitamin C, and antioxidants will work quickly to reduce fine lines and wrinkles, making you look good and young.

Let it sit for about five minutes and then rinse with warm water

Bromelain is known for smoothing skin, and it's also great for getting rid of swelling.

If you have puffy eyes, try applying some pineapple juice to a Q tip and gently rubbing it into your sockets under the eyes. Let it sit for about five minutes and then rinse.

Make sure you are gentle, as the skin under our eyes is very sensitive. And try not to pull too hard on them.

And if you decide to use pineapple juice, make sure it's 100% juice and, if possible, certified organic.

Pineapple juice is also great for sun-damaged skin.

However, remember that it is acidic, so be gentle and test on a very small part of your skin.

Try diluting a little pineapple juice with a little warm water, and then apply it to sunburn. Let it sit for about 10 minutes and then rinse slowly.

In general, it is difficult to overcome the natural healing properties of pineapple juice

Chapter 4

The acne

I am sure each of you is familiar with acne. Almost everyone has this skin disorder, right? Well, technically known as acne vulgaris, this skin disorder annually affects millions of people from different walks of life. Studies have found that most teens are the regular target of this disease, although babies and adults are also affected. It was even found that around 80 percent of teens develop acne, particularly for women.

What is acne?

According to certain studies, acne varies from mild to tremendously severe. It usually forms when the lining of the skin duct and sebaceous glands begin to work overtime. With the appearance of acne, the lining of the duct actually sheds cells that are then transported to the skin peel by sebum. Once the duct is blocked, it is when the sebum and cells begin to accumulate, forming a plug known as a comedone.

Once the plug remains below the plane of the skin, white spots or "closed comedo" occur. If the plug increases and leaves the skin duct, it is called an "open comet" or pimple since the top is dark. As you know, this is not absolutely dirt, therefore it will not wash off.

There are many factors that contribute to acne formation, but in terms of its actual cause, no one is really sure what exactly causes acne or why it starts in adolescence. However, hereditary factor tops the list. It has long been considered as the most important factor that plays an important role in the development of acne. As most people believe, if a member of your family had acne, there is a good chance that you also have acne.

Although acne is very common among teens, acne should not control your life. There are many ways to fight acne, and one of them is to maintain a healthy lifestyle.

Experts have said that when treating a person for acne, the only way to get effective treatment results is through various healthy lifestyle changes. When I say "healthy lifestyle changes," it includes the way you eat, sleep, work, play, etc. As much as possible, you should try to focus on all the areas that need change. This is very important to complete a sustained effort. If your goal is to treat your bothersome acne, try treating yourself in every possible way.

Overcome stress

One of the most common dilemmas people face is stress. Stress that is not normal. So what happens when the body becomes too stressed? Experts have found that in this case, the adrenal cortex converts adrenal androgens to the hormone testosterone in both men and women, which in turn produces overactive sebaceous glands. As discovered, women's ovaries are capable of producing 25 percent of testosterone, while 75 percent of the hormone comes from adrenal androgens.

When men's and women's bodies are stressed, more adrenal androgens are released, causing a double amount of testosterone. It is this doubling effect that makes the T-zone of the face fat, while other areas are still dry from dehydration. Also keep in mind that adult acne is sometimes the by-product of stress and dehydration. And, water and estrogen are the factors that calm the body's stress alarm system.

Some other tips to control acne

Here are other tips that have helped hundreds of people suffering from acne. Hopefully these will also help you:

Water is better

Did you know that one of the most damaging things you can do to your skin is not drinking enough water? This can quickly start to age your skin. The drier it is below the surface of your skin, the more damage it will cause to the top layer of your skin.

It is often said that the easiest way to cleanse and soften skin that is no longer dry is to drink plenty of water. Water has long been considered the most effective natural treatment or almost free treatment for any skin condition because it is alkaline, with a pH of 7.3. It prevents dehydration that is capable of producing sebum or oil from the sebaceous glands. Your skin needs water for it to work better, therefore doctors and nutritionists recommend a daily intake of between 6 and 8 glasses of water per day.

Water is by far the most effective acne treatment. The main support for this statement is the fact that the water is alkaline (pH 7.3) and can be considered as a natural treatment or an almost free acne treatment. Therefore, it is best that you drink at least eight glasses of water per day (10-12 is best). This will help your body flush out oil, debris, and toxins, and the water even helps moisten your skin by preventing your pores from clogging. Perhaps most importantly, water helps relieve stress and relaxes the body in the end, so you can sleep better. Keep in mind that water and sleep are factors that help reduce stress. Along with this, try to decrease your intake of coffees, sodas, teas, and alcohols as much as possible.

'Drink a lot of water'. This will not keep your skin moist, but it will help in the overall maintenance of your health (and in turn your skin). It may seem a little uncomfortable to some, however this is an important skin care tip.

One of the first things you will notice, without adequate hydration, are the wrinkles on your hands and arms. You will also notice dryness in and around your elbows and heels.

Also, you will see a dramatic increase in wrinkles on your face.

It is never too late to delay this process and begin to heal the damage already done. Even if you don't like water, force yourself to consume at least 64 ounces of water a day.

Avoid astringents

If your goal is to have beautiful skin, then you should try to avoid natural astringent soaps and any astringent agents that shrink your skin pores, like oatmeal, witch hazel, very cold water, and alcohol. It was actually found that when your skin pores shrink, more oils get clogged in your skin pores, causing acne to appear.

Avoid stimulants

Avoid coffee, tea, cigarettes, and excess sugar from candy and soda. It is often said that anything that can affect the entire body, brain, and nervous system can easily stimulate the sebaceous glands to release more oil. This oil has to leave the body through the pores, making your acne worse in the end. Stimulants even cause stress.

Take care of your diet

Keep in mind that diet affects acne. So be careful what you eat. As much as possible, try to eat low-fat foods, since fats produce more oils in the body that are capable of causing acne.

Avoid alcohol

Some people think that alcohol is one of the best ways to relax and relieve stress. Well, alcohol can do this, but studies have found that alcohol causes acne to form. It is considered capable of producing acne knowing that it is an astringent, therefore it reduces the pores of the skin and makes them more prone to clogging. Other than that, alcohol inhibits sleep, therefore causing more fatigue and stress, making acne worse.

Account hot and very cold

When considering baths, you should avoid hot and very cold water on acne-affected skin areas. Use warm water instead; perhaps well below 98.5 degrees on your skin.

Avoid scouring and abrasives

Washing and abrasives should be avoided. Experts have said that they irritate the skin, which should be left intact as a natural barrier against acne-causing bacteria.

Sun for beautiful skin

As you know, the sun kills bacteria, but that does not mean it will not harm the skin. Keep in mind that the sun also acts as an astringent that dries, tightens, and clogs up skin pores. Therefore, you should only spend a limited time in the sun. At least 15 minutes a day for the face and arms is enough.

Avoid extremely cold weather

If extreme heat causes clogging of the pores, extremely cold weather also causes it. Therefore, avoid extremely cold weather so as not to freeze and clog pores. It is ideal for hydrating the face and body, and staying in temperatures ranging from 70 to 80 degrees Fahrenheit.

Swimming helps

Exercise to reduce stress by swimming in a properly treated indoor pool. But, if possible, use the purified ozone pool. It is interesting to know that the pool water is typically 75 to 85 degrees Fahrenheit, which is well below the normal body temperature of 98.6 degrees. Therefore, pool water cools the entire body, including acne-affected areas, while providing excellent exercise for the rest of you. This even reduces stress and physical attention.

Think clean

You also need to change bedding, wash cloths and body towels after each use. It is because they are great places for acne-causing bacteria to grow and reapply to the skin later. Also, wash white face cloths, pillowcases, and personal underwear every day with vinegar, tea tree oil, or lime, lemon, or orange essential oils to decrease acne-related bacterial development. It is also often suggested that you apply a natural laundry detergent.

In fact, there are many ways to control and combat acne, but maintaining a healthy lifestyle is, so far, the best to consider. It is important to note that healthy lifestyles will lead to healthier skin and body. Changing your unfavorable habits will reward you with better overall health, more energy, and clearer skin to show the world. If you have ever been afraid to make changes, don't do it. Of course, the initial effects may be difficult to understand at first, but as you go along you'll discover that you can quickly learn to adapt to them.

Chapter 5

Healthy tips

Many of us are aware of the skin. We often want our skin to look young and healthy, and we really do something just to protect our skin from possible harm to our environment.

Our skin is our largest organ that performs various functions. It mainly protects us against the invasion of foreign substances and serves as a transfer point for the release of toxins from our bodies, therefore our skin is worthy of protection and care.

Now if you find yourself coveting the beautiful skin of models and celebrities in most magazines today, here are some tips to help you get beautiful skin.

Tip # 1: Watch your diet

Nutrition also plays a vital role in skin health. Specific foods, such as acidic foods and dairy products, are said to be potent in causing an allergic reaction in some people. Furthermore, one of the widely debated topics in the area of nutrition today is chocolates. Some say that chocolate affects the condition of the skin, while others say that it does not. Whatever the result, the best recommendation is to follow a nutritious diet that contains a quantity of fresh fruits and green leafy vegetables, as well as fiber.

Tip # 2: Consider exfoliants

Many experts say exfoliating your skin is another great way to achieve beautiful skin. Therefore, try to invest in a good body scrub or "loofah" as it is commonly called, as it is capable of removing dead skin cells from your body. Consequently, this should be done once or twice a week to free the skin to breathe. Additionally, scrubs help prevent ingrown hair development.

However, it is necessary to avoid the use of anybody scrub on the skin of the face. The main reason for this precaution is that facial tissue is more sensitive and finer than those of the body.

Today, there are a plethora of exfoliating sponges on the market, as well as a number of really good exfoliating gels that are specially formulated for facial skin. However, one of the necessary things to keep in mind is that people with acne-affected skin should not apply exfoliating gels or sponges, as they can aggravate the acne infection. Try to consider those exfoliating products for acne-prone skin in the form of a skin-peeling treatment. These products are now commonly offered in most of my salons anywhere in the world. And, perhaps, it's best to consider consulting a skin specialist before embarking on any form of skin.

Tip # 3: Consider a healthy routine for facial care

When it comes to facial skin care, getting into a healthy beauty routine is not a bad thing. Most doctors today strongly recommend that you cleanse, moisturize, and tone your skin twice a day. When cleaning, never stop remembering cleaning the neck area, including the face. Apply a moisturizer or neck cream afterward.

Before going to bed at night, always remember to remove all makeup. Clean your skin before bed, no matter how tired you feel. It was discovered that during the night, the skin goes through a process of elimination and cannot breathe properly if it is clogged with makeup. And you may also discover that sleeping with makeup on will make your skin "break" with blemishes.

When it comes to shaving for men, some men may experience shaving rashes. For many, these rashes lower their self-esteem, but it's not really a big problem to think about. There are many ways to avoid rashes. Perhaps one of the best is making sure that when shaving, the razor strokes follow the direction of hair growth. That's just it!

Also, scars on the face can sometimes be unpleasant. To heal a scar, it is recommended to use jasmine or neroli essential oils diluted in carrier oil. This is considered effective for removing facial scars, and even works on stretch marks as well. However, if you noticed that the scar or stretch mark has turned silver or white, please note that it can no longer be removed. And, if it is pink or red, there is a good chance it can heal.

When it comes to bruises, there are Arnica creams and ointments that are helpful in healing bruises. It is also interesting to know that one way to treat bruises quickly and effectively is to use Vicks Vaporub on the affected area.

Tip # 4: Heal your feet

When it comes to skin care, the feet are often neglected. So if you care that you haven't found time for a professional pedicure, try filling a soccer ball or bowl with warm water and adding your favorite essential oil. Soak your feet for about fifteen minutes. Then dry them and apply a rough skin remover on them. Rinse this off and dry your feet well. And, if you are considering a pedicure, simply add a little body cream to your feet for a quick and easy pedicure.

Tip # 5: Tie your bangs off your face

For many people, testing their bangs off their faces for a few hours each day is somehow necessary. Supporting this statement is the belief that it will prevent blemishes from forming on your forehead, especially if you are prone to oily hair. It is observed that sometimes these oily deposits in the hair can be transferred to the skin, which eventually causes the skin to develop acne or any disorder.

Tip # 6: Avoid Too Much Sun Exposure

One of the most common precautions when it comes to skin care is to avoid excessive sun exposure. As you know, excessive exposure to sunlight causes sunburn. So while today's sunscreens only block UVB rays and still let harmful UVA rays in, it's wise to cover up before venturing into Apollo's hands. If possible, wear a wide-brimmed hat while you care for your yard to keep the sun away from your face.

Tip # 7: exercise

In addition to considering a healthy diet, exercising your body also helps keep your skin healthy. Keep in mind that proper exercise not only keeps the body in shape by regulating oxygen; it also improves the shine of the skin as well.

Tip # 8: Get enough rest

A common problem that people face is stress; the one that is not normal it was discovered that when a person is stressed, the adrenal cortex converts adrenal androgens to the hormone testosterone in both men and women, which in turn produces overactive sebaceous glands. These adrenal androgens are released causing a double amount of testosterone, causing the face to become fat, while other areas of the body are still dry from dehydration. Therefore, taking adequate rest that includes 6 to 8 hours of restful sleep is the best way to rejuvenate your skin.

Tip # 9: Other helpful skin care tips

There are many home remedies for skin care. One of the most commonly suggested is to mix the egg white and honey well and then apply them to the face. Experts believe this smoothes the skin and helps reduce wrinkles.

Also, you should try mixing turmeric powder with milk and applying it to your face. This specifically eliminates tanning and helps reduce facial hair growth. When it is already applied to the face, rub it with a good facial scrub and then wash it off with cold water. It is not extremely cold water. You can even store it overnight.

Some experts also recommend mixing oatmeal together with curd and tomato juice for facial care. This is often kept for 20 minutes and washed with cold water. This is also powerful in eliminating tanning and keeping skin clear.

Did you know that cucumber juice is an excellent astringent for beautiful and smooth skin? Yes it is. Applying cucumber juice to the face helps tighten the pores on the skin. However, it is necessary to wash it after 15 minutes to obtain a better result.

Another great tip for conscious skin is to apply petroleum jelly to your entire body after a shower. Then bathe again after an hour and repeat this twice a month. This also improves the condition of the skin.

Finally, you can use glycolic acid (soft peel) and trichloroacetic acid (medium peel solutions. As found, these peels are safe and not overly aggressive. They do not require time off from work or social activities, and these peels soften, soften, and refresh the skin.

Always keep in mind that your skin reflects your health. It is the canvas of your body and one of your valuable assets. So for good skin care, start developing healthy habits that generally protect your valuable possession, which is the skin, from external and internal forces. Your daily habits mean it all, as it is the only skin you will get.

Healthy skin is really one of the most important ingredients to improve beauty. This article on skin care tips is an effort to bring you the top 10 best skin care tips. The list of skincare tips has been restricted to 10 because anything more than that would not only be difficult to remember, but would also hide the most important skincare tips.

* Knowing your skin type is one of the most important tips for skin care. This is important because not all skin care products fit everyone. In fact, all skin care products specify the type of skin they serve as well.

* 'Drink a lot of water'. This will not keep your skin moist, but it will help in the overall maintenance of your health (and in turn your skin). It may seem a little uncomfortable to some, however this is an important skin care tip.

* Clean your skin regularly (1-2 times a day). A very effective skin care tip that helps remove dirt and other rough elements from your skin. Cleaning is especially important when you have been away from home (and therefore exposed to contaminants, dust, etc.). This skin care tip also advocates using Luke's warm water for cleansing (hot and cold water can damage the skin).

* Be gentle, after all it's your skin. Don't rub / exfoliate too hard or too often. Similarly, don't apply too much or too many skin care products. An essential advice for skin care.

* Keep your skin moist at all times. This is one of the most important tips for skin care. Don't let your skin dry. Dryness causes the outer layer of your skin to break, giving it a rough and unattractive appearance. Use moisturizers / emollients. Moisturizers work best when applied while the skin is still wet.

* Avoid using soap on the face. Soap should only be used under the neck. A small but important advice for skin care.

* Use sunscreen to protect yourself from harmful UV radiation from the sun. You can use daytime moisturizers that have sunscreen attached. Wear them even when it's cloudy. UV radiation is known to cause skin cancer, so follow this advice for skin care without fail.

* A little exercise and a good sleep are also essential, not only for skin care but also for your overall health. Lack of sleep can cause wrinkles to form under your eyes, and lack of exercise can cause your skin to loosen. In addition, exercise and sleep also help combat stress. So, in addition to being a skin care tip, it is also a health care tip.

* Treat skin dilemmas carefully. This skin care tip tries not to ignore any skin dilemmas. Consult your dermatologist before using a skin care product (so that it does not end up further damaging your skin).

* Beat stress. Everyone knows the harmful effects of stress, however, sometimes claiming that the obvious is also essential (and therefore this skin care tip found its place here). Yes, stress also damages the skin. So, take a break or enjoy a warm bubble bath or just sleep well.

Chapter 6

Anti aging skin care

What happened this morning when you got out of bed and found yourself looking at all the wrinkles that covered your face? Did you think "Oh my god! Not only do I feel old, but I look old." This doesn't have to be such a rude shock when you apply the following anti-aging skin care tips.

2. Vitamin C and E will reduce skin aging

As you age, there are certain environmental pollutions that wreak havoc on your skin. How:

• Cigarette smoke

• Aggressive chemicals

• Vegetable herbicides

• The air pollution

• And others

Admittedly, it takes years for these things to work on the surface of your skin. However, as they work on you, they break down the living cells in your body, causing major problems under the skin. This damage affects collagen and the elasticity of your skin. This in turn will cause your skin to sag and cause more wrinkles.

You should avoid situations where you are exposed to these problems as much as possible. But you can significantly reduce damage by getting plenty of vitamin E and C. The best way to do this is to eat foods rich in those vitamins, or at least supplement your diet with vitamin E and C capsules.

3. Stay out of the sun

Excessive exposure to sunlight will cause a staggering amount of damage to your skin. A deeply tanned young body looks great and sexy. However, as you get older, sun-damaged skin will start to look like a wrinkled mess of leather.

This does not mean that you cannot go out and enjoy the outdoors. It means you must use common sense about sun exposure. You can use a sunscreen to reduce the harmful effects of the sun's ultraviolet rays.

If it does, be sure to check the time to determine how long it is effective. Most sunscreens begin to lose their protective ability once exposed to air and body chemicals. Therefore, you must be sure to reapply sunscreen to maintain proper protection.

Another side note on sun damaged skin to consider is skin damaged by the sun's ultraviolet rays; causes skin cancer. What you may not know is that skin cancer is one of the deadliest forms of cancer. It is the second after lung cancer in cancer deaths.

As you can see, the three tips are not radical at all, drink plenty of water, avoid situations that expose you to environmental pollutants, and protect yourself from the deadly ultraviolet rays of the sun. You'll be pleasantly surprised at how your skin will appear, when you use common sense and these 3 healthy anti-aging skincare tips.

Chapter 7

Good and bad habits

As everyone knows, our skin is the obvious appearance of who or what we are, or perhaps we would like to be. However, it is more than just a mask. It is the largest organ in our body, which is a complex and highly dynamic system that plays a crucial role in our general well-being. Our skin sometimes even reflects our health too. It is the canvas of our body and one of its most valuable assets.

Knowing how important our skin is, we must do something great for it. Perhaps starting a healthy habit is the most important move, as this helps our valuable possession of external and internal sources. Keep in mind that it is the only skin we have, so it is worth protecting.

Three habits to break

Is your skin as smooth and healthy as you would like? You can be sabotaging it without even knowing it. So here are three of the habits you should break as they wreak havoc on your skin. Write them down for beautiful, healthy skin.

Bad habit # 1: dry shave

It is important to note that shaving dry legs and armpits can cause irritation, ingrown hairs, and razor burns. Therefore, to nourish the skin, it is worth considering softening it in the shower for about 10 minutes. Most experts even recommend these things for those who want to get attractive skin. After doing so, you should apply a layer of shaving cream and not soap, which will dull the shaver and invite cuts. You should shave in long strokes. And, apply a body lotion after showering.

Bad habit # 2: ignoring incidental sun exposure

Admittedly, walking from your car or wherever you are to the office in the sun may not be as harmful as spending hours cooking on the beach. However, it is important to note that even a few minutes of exposure here and there does not mean that you will not have wrinkles. It does bring wrinkles the same way. For that, you should try using a daily SPF lotion specially formulated for facial application. Many experts suggest brands of SPF lotions like Clinique and Neutrogena, as they have versions that really work well under makeup.

Bad habit # 3: avoid exfoliation

Considering exfoliation of the skin is often said to produce excellent results. Perhaps this is because if you ignore exfoliation, dead skin cells will start to accumulate on the skin, causing itching and rashes, especially in unpredictable or dry weather. Therefore, it is often recommended that you rub your skin daily with a puff, loofah, or grainy scrub to help sweep away rough skin. After scrubbing, apply moisturizer to maintain smoothness.

Nine habits to maintain

Now that you know about the three bad habits to break, now is the time to consider what habits should be kept to covet the most attractive skin on earth. Most dermatologists share the following habits as their best tips for a fair complexion. So if you want your skin to be on your behavior, you need to change your acting now for the better and follow some rules.

Good habit # 1: avoid too many cosmeceuticals

Numerous experts have said that with more and more beauty potions with alpha-hydroxy acids (AHAs), antioxidants, salicylic acids, and retinoids in them, mix a cleanser from one line with a scrub or daytime moisturizer from another, then a night cream from still another can cause over exfoliation and irritation. Without a doubt, this can add up to a real dilemma, especially for those women who have dark and olive complexions. This is also possible for women who are more prone to discoloration when their skin is irritated.

So to be really safe, it's important that you only stick with one product line. But, just use the line of products that are formulated to work together. It is often said that if, for example, you use prescription products like the famous Renova, the advice of your dermatologist is very necessary. Ask your specialist about mixing prescription treatments with over-the-counter cosmeceuticals. Just don't overdo beauty products.

Good habit # 2: consider healthy exercise

Exercise is ideal for beautiful skin. Therefore, it is worth trying at least twenty to thirty minutes of any aerobic exercise. It will give it a shine, as it is often said. One of the supports for this is the fact that exercise increases blood flow. It is this increased blood flow that will bring more nutrients to the skin. However, it is important to note that sebum or oil buildup through perspiration can lead to sweat band acne, folliculitis, and stinging heat. But do not worry: there is a simple solution to this: shower as soon as possible after shaking the loot.

Good habit # 3: Intimate with the phone? Do not be!

Always keep in mind that constant rubbing on the mouthpiece can cause rashes around the chin and mouth. This is what many people have believed, including dermatologists. Therefore, it is important that when talking to someone on the phone, you keep the phone away from the areas mentioned when speaking. Also, clean the phone frequently with a mild soapy solution or perhaps with alcohol.

Good habit # 4: Examine your birthday outfit for stains

When it comes to skin care, any sudden or suspicious mole, bump, or other growth on the skin is a reason to see a dermatologist. However, as skin cancer rates skyrocketed, having a full body checkup by a professional is very crucial. This is especially true for those of us who live in the generation of baby sunscreen with oil and iodine.

Also, those in a high-risk group, which means having a personal or family history of skin cancer, lots of moles, light skin, or light eyes or hair, are said to see a specialist for a regular checkup. The regular exam should begin in adolescence and probably no later than age 35. However, even if you do not belong to a high risk group, it is recommended that between the ages of 20 and 40, people should have a cancer related checkup. The checkup should include a skin exam and should be considered every three to four years. Once you turn 40, start having a cancer-related exam with a skin exam every year. Other than that,

Good Habit # 5: Eat Healthy Foods

Healthy foods refer to those that help your skin and body fight bad external and internal forces. You should consider antioxidants such as vitamins A, C, and E, as they are very powerful for sun damage and fight certain types of cancer, including skin cancer. This is actually the reason that antioxidants are essential to your health. Along with this, a well-balanced diet is recommended. This means being comfortable with a diet that contains at least five daily servings of fruits and vegetables, plus a multivitamin that meets RDA standards.

Good habit # 6: Avoid wearing your makeup in bed at night

I guess you all know this rule, but sometimes you do it anyway. Well, you need to keep in mind that the undercoats, powder, and even blusher left overnight can clog your skin pores and lead to acne or folliculitis. Knowing this warning, you should remove it before bedtime. You can do this by using a mild cleaner without soap. However, remember not to waste money on a cleaner with glycolic acid or AHA. As they say, it is not on the face long enough to absorb into the skin. The mentioned ingredients are more effective in humectants than in cleansers.

Good habit # 7: Hands off those pimples

We all have pimples. That's the truth. But, that doesn't mean we will let those pimples ruin our lives. We must do something to prevent them from forming, and we must do it simply so as not to puncture, puncture, burst or squeeze them. These actions can prolong the life of a grain and worsen the problem. They can even cause scarring and spread of infection. Therefore, to speed healing, never squeeze or pinch. Simply wipe your face, and then apply a warm compress, such as a clean, damp cloth. Then apply an over-the-counter cream or lotion that contains a drying agent such as salicylic acid, benzoyl peroxide, or sulfur.

Good habit # 8: get enough rest and sleep

Many of us do not get enough sleep and are stressed. Actually, there have been no conclusive studies on how tiredness affects the skin condition. But, the effects are generally not difficult to detect. One of the most common effects is circles under the eyes. Therefore, to avoid any unfavorable effects that may occur, you should budget for sleep time. This can include a short nap every time you can handle it. However, do not sleep in the same position for years, as this can lead to wrinkles. Perhaps the best way to consider is to find a special pillow that helps prevent sleep wrinkles on your face.

Good habit # 9: Drink plenty of water

The bottom line here is to adopt plenty of water every day as your mantra. You should know that drinking water keeps you hydrated. This even helps your skin look and feel better. Therefore, get the standard 6 to 8 eight-ounce glasses throughout the day. You can drink more if you exercise a lot. And, if you like low-calorie liquids, drink more water to avoid dehydration. Keep in mind that most new sugar substitutes today are dehydrating.

As presented, there are many habits that we often ignore, thinking that they do not play an important role in our lives. But the truth is that everything we do has a corresponding meaning and role that must be revealed and considered. If your main goal is to achieve beautiful skin and general well-being, it is worth maintaining a healthy lifestyle. Keep in mind that our daily habits are everything.

Chapter 8

Herbal skin care

Skincare is not a recent issue; it has been in practice since ancient times, when herbal skin care was probably the only way to take care of your skin. However, skincare has been transformed in a big way. Herbal skincare routines have been replaced by chemical / synthetic based skincare routines. Herbal skin care recipes that used to be commonplace today are not that popular (and even unknown to a large population). This transformation from herbal to synthetic skin care can probably be attributed to two things: our laziness (or just the fast pace of life) and the commercialization of skin care. Herbal skin care products have even been marketed. These commercial herbal skin care products must be mixed with preservatives to increase their shelf life, making them less effective than fresh, homemade ones. However, it seems that things are changing rapidly and more and more people are choosing natural and herbal skin care routines. But still, none want to make them at home, and therefore the commercial market for herbal skin care products is on the rise. It seems that things are changing rapidly and more and more people are choosing natural and herbal skin care routines. But still, none want to make them at home, and therefore the commercial market for herbal skin care products is on the rise. It seems that things are changing rapidly and more and more people are choosing natural and herbal skin care routines. But still, none want to make them at home, and therefore the commercial market for herbal skin care products is on the rise.

So what are these herbs or herbal skin care mechanisms?

Aloe vera, which is an extract from the aloe plant, is one of the best examples of herbal skin care products. Freshly extracted aloe vera is a natural hydrant that helps calm skin. It also helps heal cuts and treat sunburn.

Various herbs are known to have cleansing properties. Dandelion, chamomile, lime blossoms, and rosemary herbs are some examples of these cleansers. Its herbal skin care properties are invoked when combined with other herbs such as tea.

Antiseptics are another important part of herbal skin care. Lavender, marigold, thyme, and fennel are good examples of herbs that have antiseptic properties. Lavender water and rose water also make good tonics.

Tea plays an important role in herbal skin care. Tea extracts are used to treat skin that has been damaged by UV radiation.

Oils prepared from herbal extracts present another herbal skincare means. Tea tree oil, lavender oil, borage oil, and evening primrose oil are some popular oils used in herbal skin care. Some fruit oils (eg, Fruit Extracts like Banana, Apple, and Melon) are used in bath gels (as a hydrating blend)

Homeopathic treatments and aromatherapy are also under the umbrella of herbal skin care remedies.

Herbal skin care is good not only for routine skin nutrition but also for treating skin disorders like eczema and psoriasis. Most herbal skin care products have no side effects (the most important reason for preferring them to synthetic products). Also, herbal skin care products can be easily prepared at home, making them even more attractive. Therefore, herbal skin care is the way to go. However, this does not mean that you completely discard synthetic products. Some people go to the point of debating with their dermatologist whether he / she suggests a synthetic product.

Chapter 9

Lotions versus creams for skin care

There is no shortage of creams and lotions for skin care on the market. Name an ailment and you will find hundreds of creams, lotions, and other skin care products. As a result of ongoing research and due to increasing demand, the number of skin care products appears to be on the rise. Skincare lotions and skincare creams are the most popular ways these products are available, and there always seems to be a debate about which shape is best.

Well, there is no definitive answer to this. It seems more a matter of personal choice. However, fatty creams are surely less popular compared to non-greasy (or less greasy) ones. Since the application of skin care creams is easier, they appear to be preferred (rather than lotions) in cases where the skin care product should not be removed immediately after application. Therefore, skin care creams seem more popular as moisturizers than as cleansers or toners. For toners, lotions seem to be preferred over skin care creams. There are some skin care creams that also act as toners, but in general toners are available only in liquid form. For cleaning, lotions and creams for skin care are equally popular; however, the inclination seems more towards lotions.

Creams are known to be more effective at keeping skin moist; therefore, the most popular form of skin care creams are moisturizers. For the same reason, many people tend to associate skin care creams with dry, sensitive skin. Although true to some extent, skin care creams are not only used for dry skin, but are also used to make products for oily skin, for example vitamin A creams and sulfur creams that help to reduce the rate of sebum production.

Skin care creams are also used for products that adapt to skin disorders, especially for disorders that require application of the product in a small local area. This is again due to the fact that skin care creams are easier to apply (no waste) to the affected area. However, in cases where the skin needs to be washed using a medication / product, the lotion is a better option. Primarily, manufacturers are also aware of this fact, making it easier to choose between a lotion and a skin care cream.

Eye creams and anti-aging creams are other examples where skin care cream is preferred over its lotion counterpart.

Whatever your choice (cream or lotion), knowing how to use it effectively is more important than anything else.

Chapter 10

Organic skin care

"If it can be done naturally, why choose artificial means?" This is the basic premise on which 'organic skin care' works. Organic skin care is the most natural form of 'skin care'. In fact, "organic skin care" was probably the first to be used by man when he first woke up to the needs of his skin. 'Organic skin care' is not only more skin friendly, it is also inexpensive. If exercised the right way, organic skin care can prevent many skin disorders from developing and can help keep your skin healthy and young for much longer.

Organic fruits and vegetables are the most popular things in organic skin care routines, for example cucumber is very common in organic skin care routines. Turmeric, apple, papaya, ginger are others that find wide use in organic skincare routines. These organic materials have a very refreshing and vitalizing effect on your skin. Almost all skin care books / guides have a section on organic skin care (including the actions of various fruits and vegetables on the skin). So, pick the ones that are best suited for your skin type and start experimenting with them until you finally select the ones that are best suited for inclusion in your organic skincare routine. It is important that you use fresh organic fruits / vegetables. Do not try to use the rotten ones for your skin, their only place is the garbage can.

Milk is known to have good cleaning properties; in fact, the name of some skin care products contains the word 'milk' on them. A combination of milk and ground oats acts as a wonderful cleanser.

Ground oats are especially good for oily skin and are a popular ingredient in the organic skin care regimen. It is used in various combinations, for example with egg, honey, milk and fruit, for the preparation of organic facial packages.

Wheat germ is another ingredient in organic skin care procedures. It is rich in vitamin E and is known for its exfoliation and moisturizing properties. Wheat germ, in various combinations with other organic materials, is used to prepare facial masks for normal and dry skin. Wheat germ oil is another way to use wheat germ for organic skin care.

Yogurt and sour cream are other organic materials that are popular for their exfoliating and moisturizing properties.

The use of organic honey is also popular in organic skin care procedures. Helps retain moisture and helps impart a shiny appearance to the skin.

Rose water takes its place as a toner in organic skincare routines. Lavender water is also popular.

'Organic skin care' uses combinations of various organic materials that complement each other and improve the effectiveness of each. Furthermore, these combinations are also useful to overcome the harmful effects (if any) of various organic materials that form them.

Organic skin care is truly an art that, once perfected, can yield wonderful results in a very cost-effective way.

Chapter 11

"Personal skin care" is a routine

We all know the importance of "personal skin care". Opinion on how to do it (for personal skin care) differs from person to person. Some people believe that going to beauty salons every other day is personal skin care. Others believe that personal skin care is just a matter of applying a little cream or lotion to the skin, from time to time. Then there are people who think that personal skin care is an event that happens once a month or once a year. Still others dealt with 'personal skin care' all the time. However, personal skin care is not that complicated and also not that expensive (considering how beneficial it is). Personal skin care follows a routine or procedure to meet the needs of your skin.

Even before starting a routine, you need to determine your skin type (oily, dry, sensitive, normal, etc.) and select the right personal skin care products (you may have to experiment with some personal skin care products). Skin care). Here is a routine that should work for most people with normal skin.

The first thing in the personal routine of skin care is 'Cleaning'. The three main ingredients in a cleaner are oil, water, and surfactants (wetting agents). Oil and surfactants remove dirt and oil from the skin and water, then expel it and cleanse the skin. You may have to try a couple of cleaners before you find the one that works best for you. However, you should always use soap-free cleansers. Also, you should use lukewarm Luke water for cleaning (cold and hot water can both harm your skin). Be careful not to over-clean your skin and end up damaging your skin in the process.

The second thing in your personal skincare routine is exfoliation. The skin follows a natural maintenance process in which it removes dead cells and replaces them with new skin cells. Exfoliation is just one way to ease the skin in this process. Dead skin cells are not able to respond to personal skin care products, but they still consume these products, preventing them from reaching new skin cells. Therefore, removing dead skin cells is important to increase the effectiveness of all personal skin care products. In general, the exfoliation is carried out just after cleaning. As with any personal skin care procedure, it is important that you understand how much exfoliation you need. Exfoliate 4-5 times per week for oily / normal skin and 1-2 times per week for dry / sensitive skin. Exfoliate a few more times in hot, humid climates.

Next in your personal skin care routine are moisturizers. This is one of the most important things in personal skin care. Even people with oily skin need moisturizers. Moisturizers not only seal moisture in skin cells, but also attract it (from the air) whenever necessary. However, using too much moisturizer can clog your skin pores and end up damaging your skin. The amount of moisturizer your skin needs will become apparent within a week of using the moisturizer. Also, applying the moisturizer is best when the skin is still wet.

The latest in the routine of personal skin care is sunscreen. Many moisturizers (daytime moisturizers / creams) come with UV protection, so you can reap double the benefits. Such moisturizers are recommended for every day (regardless of whether it's sunny or cloudy).

Again, experiment with various personal skin care products as well as how much you need to apply. What works best for you is the best personal skin care recipe for you. However, if you have any type of skin dilemma, it is best to consult your dermatologist before starting to use any personal skin care product.

Chapter 12

Serious skin care

"Serious skin care" is about maintaining healthy, radiant skin throughout your life. As you get older, your body's natural skin care mechanisms weaken. Therefore, "serious skin care" is about responding to the changing needs of your skin. Therefore, "serious skin care" is constantly evaluating, analyzing, and changing your skin care routines. Your skincare routine should change based on environmental conditions, your age, and changes in your skin type.

"Serious skin care" is also about awareness. With technological advances and research, more and more facts come to light every day. Also, the composition and nature of skin care products seem to be changing over time. Therefore, trying new products is also part of serious skin care. However, 'serious skincare' recommends using a new product on a small (non-facial) patch of skin first, just to see how your skin reacts.

'Serious skincare' also means knowing how to use your skincare products. Good practices include things like applying moisturizers while the skin is wet, using upward strokes for better penetration of skin care products, removing makeup before bed, cleaning before moisturizing, or applying makeup, using the correct amount of skin care products etc. Therefore, increasing the effectiveness of your skincare products is another focus area of serious skincare.

Some precautions, such as avoiding contact with detergents, are also part of serious skin care. 'Serious skin care' means being kind to your skin. Things like excessive exfoliation, the use of low-quality products and the application of strong chemicals are harmful to the skin. Some people have a misconception about serious skin care. For them, serious skin care is using large amounts of products as often as possible. However, this really isn't serious skincare (and that's why awareness is so important).

"Serious skin care" is also about visiting your dermatologist for the treatment of skin disorders. Ignoring skin disorders can be fatal to your skin and can lead to permanent damage. Therefore, if things don't improve with over-the-counter medications, you should immediately visit a dermatologist. Self-surgery, for example, squeezing acne / pimples is a big no-no (it can lead to permanent skin damage).

Therefore, serious skin care is more about precautions and preventive measures (than treatment). Serious skin care is about being proactive and reactive. In fact, we can say that "serious skin care" is about being proactive about your skin's needs so that the need to be reactive is minimized.

Chapter 13

The Facts about Oily Skin Care

To start the discussion about caring for oily skin, it is imperative to first understand the cause behind oily skin. Simply put, oily skin is the result of excessive sebum production (a fatty substance naturally produced by the skin). As everyone knows, the excess of everything is bad; so excessive sebum is also bad. It leads to clogging of the skin pores, resulting in the accumulation of dead cells and thus the formation of pimples / acne. In addition, oily skin also spoils your appearance. Therefore, "oily skin care" is as important as "skin care" for other skin types.

The basic goal of "oily skin care" is to remove excess sebum or oil from the skin. However, oily skin care procedures should not lead to complete removal of the oil. "Oily skin care" begins with the use of a cleanser. However, not all cleaners will work. You need a cleanser that contains salicylic acid, that is, a beta-hydroxy acid that slows the rate of sebum production. Cleaning should be done twice a day (and even more in hot and humid conditions).

Most oily skin care products do not contain oil; however, it is always good to check the ingredients of the product, before buying it. This is especially important if a product is marked "suitable for all skin types" rather than "oily skin care product". 'Oily skin care' also depends on the degree of fat, if it is not too oily, so some of these 'fit for all' products might work for you, too. For extremely oily skin, only oily skin care products are suitable. Your oily skin care routine may include an alcohol-based toner (for extremely oily skin). This may be the second step in your oily skin care routine, i.e. right after cleaning. However, excessive toning can harm your skin.

The next step in your oily skin care routine can be a mild moisturizer. Again, the degree of oil on your skin will determine if you need to include this in your oily skin care routine. If you decide to include a moisturizer, be sure to use one that is oil, wax and lipid free.

You could also use a clay mask (for example, once a week) as a measure for oily skin care.

As for oily skin care products, you may need to try a few before you get to the one that's really right for your skin.

In case these measures do not give you the desired result, consult a good dermatologist for advice. You could prescribe stronger oily skin care products like vitamin a creams, retinoids, sulfur creams, etc. that can help counteract oily skin problems.

Chapter 14

The recipe for caring for dry skin.

Dry skin cannot be ignored. Dry skin causes cracks in the top layer of skin and makes it look really bad. The main causes of dry skin include: dry weather, hormonal changes, too much exfoliation, and treatment of other skin disorders. Also, dryness could be the inherent nature of the skin. Whatever the cause, "dry skin care" is very important (but not very difficult).

'Dry skin care' starts with moisturizers, the most effective remedy for dry skin. Moisturizers are generally classified into 2 categories based on how they provide "dry skin care".

The first category includes moisturizers that provide 'dry skin care' simply by preserving moisture within the skin, for example petrolatum. These moisturizers are relatively inexpensive and readily available (even at grocery stores).

The second category includes moisturizers that work by removing moisture from the environment and supplying it to the skin. This is a very effective way of 'dry skin care' in wet conditions. Moisturizers that provide 'dry skin care' in this way are also called moisturizers. For proper care of dry skin, you should use a non-greasy type of moisturizer, whenever possible. Moisturizers fall into this category. The ingredients of humectants include propylene glycol, urea, glycerin, hyaluronic acid, etc.

'Dry skin care' is not just about using moisturizers but also about using them properly. The best "dry skin care procedure" is to cleanse the skin before applying the moisturizer. You can make your 'dry skin care' even more effective by applying the moisturizer while the skin is still wet (after cleansing). Also, be sure to use soap-free products (especially on the face, neck, and arms). Exfoliation helps in the care of dry skin, by removing dead skin cells. However, don't exfoliate too hard. Your dry skin care procedures / products should also take care of sun protection. Avoid excessive and direct exposure to the sun (simply by using an umbrella / hat, etc.). Use a good sunscreen lotion before going out. Many moisturizers also provide sun protection, along with caring for dry skin.

It also has natural products for "dry skin care", that is, products that provide "dry skin care" naturally (without the use of synthetic chemicals). These dry skin care products provide lipid enhancements to the skin, allowing moisture retention within the skin. Another important thing for "dry skin care" is the temperature of the water you use to shower or wash your face: use warm water; too hot or too cold water can also cause dryness.

"Dry skin care" is also about being skin friendly. You should avoid strong detergents and alcohol-based cleaners. Also, after a face wash, don't rub the towel on your face, just pat gently to soak up the water.

In general, caring for dry skin is really simple for anyone who takes it seriously.

Chapter 15

Preparing your skin for the summer

We all know that dreaded feeling of wanting to wear a perfect summer before the summer hits. We all have equally good intentions: exercising, waxing our legs, preparing our shopping list of moisturizing sunscreens, and perhaps losing a few pounds.

While all of those good intentions are great, it may take a bit of work to really get ready for healthy, attractive summer skin long before summer comes.

Preparation is really key to preparing your skin for summer. No one can expect to wake up on a July morning and magically have the shiny summer skin they always dreamed of.

A little spring cleaning for your skin

When spring comes, it is important to take a good look at your cosmetics. Chances are, you're using what is left over from your winter inventory. Take a look at your moisturizer. Maybe it's time to replace that moisturizer with any of these:

* A tinted moisturizer

* A sunscreen that contains moisturizer

Next, take a look at your skin. Has being indoors created a dry, dull appearance? Start by buying or making all-natural facial cleansers at home that contain things like cucumber and / or sea salt. These things will prepare your skin as you cleanse it while you wait for summer.

Check your cosmetic colors too. In general, many women use winter colors that are slightly heavier and darker than they would during the summer months. See what needs to be replaced or, better yet, what needs to be recreated.

Light summer makeup in corals and pinks are wonderful summer options. More natural is better when it comes to summer makeup.

Increase your water intake now so that when summer comes, you won't overdo your hydration techniques.

Sun and your skin now

Start by going out in the sun for a few minutes each day, either during lunch or taking a walk all morning before taking a bath.

Of course, every time you go out in the sun, it is important to use sunscreen. A sunscreen with moisturizer is even better.

Also, be sure to buy the right glasses and hats so it won't be too soon. Starting with a little sun every day gives your skin a chance to get used to the sun once more after a long, hard winter.

This will provide an excellent foundation for your summer tan.

By priming your skin a little every day, it gives your skin a healthy, beautiful, and radiant appearance before summer begins.

How to create stunning summer skin with natural body scrubs

It is always a pleasure to have soft and sensual skin, but even more so in the summer heat. Summer is when it shows the most amount of skin and knowing that it is soft since summer is a great feeling.

Having smooth, summery skin is not only a wonderful feeling, but the process of achieving smooth, summery skin is also wonderful. Every time you do a facial or body treatment, it is a wonderful feeling of indulgence. Also, who doesn't need a little feeling of indulgence from time to time?

One of the best ways to exfoliate your body skin is, of course, with a salty body scrub. Sea salt has become extremely popular for this purpose. This is what you need to make yours.

Sea salt body scrub

Will need:

* ¾ cup of sea salt

* ¼ cup coconut oil

* 6 to 8 drops of essential oils

Mix the coconut oil with the sea salt until it forms a paste-like substance. Add the essential oil of your choice as a fragrance.

Sugar Body Scrub

* ¾ cup brown sugar

* ¼ cup sesame oil

* 6 to 8 drops of essential oil of your choice

* A ripe avocado

Peel and remove the pit from an overripe avocado. Mix the sesame oil and brown sugar with the avocado in your blender. Add essential oils once you have transferred the mixed mixture to a bowl.

Once any of these mixtures is well mixed, spread it over all the legs, making sure to pay special attention to the knees and heels of the feet. You can also use a pumice stone to scrape away dead skin from these areas.

These scrubs are also great for the knees and hands. Always secure a small area to make sure there is no allergy or irritation before putting sugar or salt scrubs mixed with essential oils anywhere on your body.

Many ingredients can be mixed and matched with your own body scrubs. For example:

* Refined sugar

* Brown sugar

* Sea salt

* Kosher salt

* Essential oils like sesame oil, vitamin E oil, lavender oil

* Honey, avocado, kiwi, coconut milk.

Once you know your body and what it is not sensitive to, the world is your oyster when it comes to natural and homemade body scrubs.

Experimenting with homemade body scrubs in the summer gives you more options than you could in the winter. Explore, enjoy, and have fun finding the perfect summer body scrub for you.

How to keep your feet alert in summer

Just as you are aware of preventing your skin from burning and staying hydrated, it is important not to neglect your feet. Your feet are beaten in the summer. Many times your feet are locked in shoes all day without much chance of breathing. Alternatively, you can spend a lot of downtime in your flip flops, and your feet can be worn and rough from all flip flops.

Keeping your feet on your toes is a great way to keep the rest of your body aligned, too.

Healthy feet mean a happy body

There are many ways to keep your feet healthy. Remember, it is your feet that carry you throughout your day and your life and we should all be nice to them.

* Natural foot scrub: Take 1/8 teaspoon of lavender mixed with 2 tablespoons of olive oil and 1 cup of kosher salt. Mix well. You can add more olive oil if necessary. Place the scrub on your feet, especially focusing on the heels. Rub well for several minutes, rinsing with warm water.

* Sweet Sugary Foot Scrub: Take ¼ cup of sugar, 15 drops of eucalyptus oil, ¼ cup of almond oil and some of your favorite moisturizers if you like. Mix well and spread on all feet. Don't forget between your toes and focus on the heels that take the most hits. Rinse well with a foot soak first and then in the shower or bathtub.

* Foot Shake: Mix oats, olive oil, baking soda, and water to form a paste that will give your wounded warriors a lot of moisture. Simply spread the paste all over your feet, rinse well, and pat dry. Put on moisturizer and cotton socks overnight and your feet will feel soft in the morning.

Soak your feet

Sometimes, you may not be in the mood or you may not have time to do a full foot scrub, so soaking tired feet is good enough.

* Add ½ cup baking soda and ½ cup Epsom salts to a bowl of very warm water. Soak your feet as long as you want. You will notice that your feet will be instantly rejuvenated and refreshed.

* A combination of milk, warm water and a little baby oil is perfect to calm and hydrate the feet.

* Eucalyptus oil, warm water, and baking soda also make a soothing and stimulating foot scrub.

Keeping feet happy and healthy is an essential form of skincare during the summer. The term hitting the pavement really applies in the summer heat like sand, walking barefoot, and the repetitive movement of flip flops and sandals taking their toll on the skin of your feet.

Keeping the skin of your feet happy and healthy keeps that bounce full of life in your wake during the foggy summer days.

Summer Essentials: Inside Out

While it's important to do skin self-exams and wear sunscreen, hats, and glasses during the summer months, it's just as essential to hydrate your skin from the inside.

Eating the right foods and drinking the right things is essential for healthy skin that glows from the inside out.

Summer is a time filled with delicious fresh fruits and vegetables, many of which are filled with hydrating water. When your body is hydrated, your skin will reflect well beyond sunscreen and shade.

Hydrating Fruits and Vegetables

* Watermelon is an excellent example of a summer fruit that hydrates. Watermelon is capable of hydrating you and your skin for a long time. It is primarily made up of water, you guessed it, and contains sodium, magnesium, and potassium. Perfect to hydrate yourself.

* Melon is full of hydration and offers Vitamin A, Vitamin C, and Potassium.

* Grapefruit: juicy, spicy and full of moisturizing juices, grapefruit is an excellent moisturizer for your skin.

* Celery: Celery is a great snack or an intermediate dish for when you want to eat something healthy. Packed with water, it also contains vitamins and mineral salts to keep the body hydrated and skin radiant.

* Strawberries: Strawberries are rich in antioxidants, but they are also great for detoxification, as are blueberries and cherries.

* Cucumbers are primarily made up of water and contain Vitamin C. Cucumbers are naturally hydrating and perfect for summer salads.

Hydrating your skin through drinks

The hotter it is, the more water you should drink. For those who don't like the taste of water, adding lemon or lime, or both, to your water can make a difference in whether or not your skin is hydrated.

Plus, brewing your own homemade fresh green tea, chilling it, and serving it with ice and lemon is a great way to hydrate that also tastes good. Adding a sprig of mint makes it the perfect hydrating drink for summer.

For many women, putting something on the outside of their face seems like the logical way to keep their skin hydrated. However, what you do inside first will always make the most difference.

Eating your summer fruits and vegetables and hydrating yourself with water and teas will not only keep your body working properly; it will also keep your skin shiny like the sun without all the side effects.

Summer facials that will make your skin sizzle

Summer is the optimal time of year to load fresh fruits and vegetables. It is also a good time to treat your skin with an all-natural, homemade facial or body scrub.

Fruits and vegetables, especially those that come out in the summer, are wonderful for providing antioxidants to the skin, hydrating, tightening skin pores, and even preventing and treating acne.

Here is a sample of the different ways you can use summer fruits and vegetables. Depending on how sensitive your skin is, it would be wise to try some of the facial recipes and see how your skin responds.

Daily apple face mask

Whether you wear this mask once a week or once a day is of course up to you.

Will need:

* Two apples

* Two tablespoons of coconut water

* Camomile tea

Peel and mash the apples and remove the seeds. Add the coconut water and enough chamomile tea so that it is forming a pasty application. Apply this to your skin that is clean and mask-ready.

Leave it on for about 10 minutes and then rinse it off with lukewarm water. Apply a cold water facial cloth to your face to close your pores. This facial should give you results of a clean, hydrated and well-toned face.

Kiwi / Strawberry Honey Facial

This mask is a great way to use fruit that is starting to overripe. If you are old school and can't stand throwing anything, this facial is perfect for you. Will need:

* Four to six overripe strawberries

* 1 overripe kiwi

* Two tablespoons of honey (the best is organic, but the normal brand is also fine)

* Two spoons of sugar

Remove the stems from the strawberries and cut them in half. Peel the kiwi, leaving the seeds as they are. The seeds will act as a scrub, so use all of the kiwi. Cut the kiwi into quarters. Put them in the blender or use a potato masher. Add the sugar. Blend until you get a creamy, soft but messy mixture.

Put the mixture on your face, which of course has no makeup and is clean. If you have an old towel to put around your neck, that would be fine as it's a very messy (but productive) facial!

Spread around your skin in circular motions. This mask is intended to exfoliate and not necessarily "stay". Once you have cleaned your entire face with this mixture, rinse with warm water.

You will feel a tingling sensation that tells you that the acidity of this fruit will work to clean your pores. The sugar exfoliates while the honey covers any irritation that may exist.

Summer fruit is great to eat, but also great for facials!

Summer skin: itching, burns and stings

While summer comes with lots of fun moments on the beach, summer nights in the backyard, and lots of time outdoors during the day, it also includes bug bites, bee stings, and sometimes some sunburn.

There are steps you can take to prevent this from happening, as well as steps you can take once they happen. And of course if it's summer these things are very likely to happen.

Dealing with insect bites

The insects are in their glory during the summer. Bees buzz and mosquitoes blink here, there, and everywhere. Fortunately, there are some creative and natural ways to avoid these creatures and treat their bites, too.

Here are some great ways to relieve the itch and burn from a mosquito bite:

* Baking Soda and Water - Baking soda has many uses, from cleaning to insect bites, and is especially wonderful for treating mosquito bites. Just make a paste of baking soda and water and apply it to the bite, and the itchiness and burning should go away pretty quickly.

* Aloe vera: Aloe vera juice or ointment directly from the aloe vera plant should be enough to alleviate the itchiness associated with a mosquito bite.

* Apple Cider Vinegar: Apple cider vinegar is ideal for relieving itching almost immediately. Apply directly to the irritated area.

Bee stings are never fun, especially for those unfortunate enough to be allergic to them. However, for those who are not allergic, there are some natural ways to treat a bee sting.

* Tea tree oil is excellent in relieving burns and pain, as well as any itching associated with a bee sting.

* Crushed aspirin mixed with water is another wonderful way to ease the pain of a bee sting. It may sound like an old wife's tale, but it really helps.

* Some people even take a small dose of an antihistamine to relieve swelling. Of course, don't take anything without checking with your doctor first.

Sunburn treatment

The best way to treat sunburn is to never have it in the first place. An ounce of prevention is worth a pound of cure, as the old saying goes.

* We recommend using sunscreen with an SPF higher than 15. We also recommend using sunscreen a few days, every day, before a tropical vacation.

* A soaking in the bath with baking soda is a great way to relieve burns and sunburn irritation.

* Tea tree oil is an excellent remedy for sunburn, as it soothes and moisturizes the skin at the same time.

It is important to remember that feeling good in the summer is as important as looking good in the summer. Take care of your skin and it will take care of you.

Summer sun: protect yourself everywhere

Almost everyone loves a good day at the beach; however, no one enjoys the results of sunburn. While sunburns are serious in themselves, skin cancer resulting from inattention in the sun could be fatal.

This is why it is so important to make sure that you and your loved ones are protected. Protecting your face is only part of the regimen. Summer sun protection for your body and even your eyes is essential.

There are many ways to protect yourself everywhere:

Protecting your face from the sun

Using an SPF of 15 or higher is the best protection for your facial skin. SPF stands for sun protection factor, which is an indication of how well a product will work to protect your skin from the sun. The higher the Skin Protection Factor, the more protection you will get.

It is also important not to use tanning oils on the facial skin. Tanning oils will attract the sun to your face and will not protect you. Also tanning oils will likely cause acne breakouts. There are many cosmetic lines that provide moisturizers along with sunscreen ranging from moderate to more expensive. Look at these products and see if you can get samples to discern which ones are best for you.

Protecting the rest of your body from the sun

While wearing a bikini can be attractive (if you're lucky enough to be able to do it!), the more skin you cover from the sun, the better off you'll be. Skin cancer is found in many areas of the body, not just the face. Covering more skin and protecting it from the dangerous ultraviolet rays of the sun makes common sense.

Beautiful Skin

Wearing a skimpy swimsuit can make you feel sexier, but the end result could be serious. Covering up is just one way to deter serious sun damage. Taking breaks is also another great way to avoid sunburn or skin cancer.

Taking a little time to sunbathe is fine if you're well protected with high-value SPF sunscreen and covering yourself. However, taking breaks under an umbrella is just as important.

Other tips to stay safe in the sun

* Don't forget to protect your eyes: sunglasses are a must.

* Don't be shy to try on a hat, you never know, you might like how it looks.

* Wear waterproof sunscreen for swimming - the sun draws in the water and can burn very easily without realizing it while having fun in the waves or in the pool.

With a little common sense, you can have fun in the sun while protecting yourself at the same time.

The importance of skin self-exams, especially during and after summer

It is essential that you self-examine your skin at various points throughout the year. However, it is very important that you monitor any changes in your skin during the summer and right after.

When the season changes and we are faced with being outdoors more often, maintaining skin care should be the most important thing on our mind. Even if you are at an outdoor barbecue and the sun is high in the sky, just because you are not wearing your bathing suit and on the beach does not mean you are not at risk.

If you have pre-existing moles or are prone to freckles, it is imperative to be aware of any changes in shape, size, or color.

How to start skin self-exams

1. First start by getting to know your body; pay attention to moles, freckles and spots.

2. Observe these things and become familiar with them. Notice the different features.

3. Look closely in a full-length mirror to check your skin from head to toe.

4. Using a smaller hand mirror, also check your back and neck.

5. Check your skin every six to eight weeks and note any changes. Any changes you see are something that should get your doctor's attention.

The importance of self-examination of the skin can be forgotten, since most people do not think to check their own skin from time to time to monitor changes. However, the potential to detect and treat skin cancer early is significant if you do a regular skin self-exam.

As with any type of cancer, early detection is key.

Continuous self-examination of the skin

It is important to continue skin self-exams every six to eight weeks and, most importantly, during the summer months.

If you notice any changes in your moles or freckles or any part of your skin that looks or feels different from your initial exam, contact your doctor as soon as possible.

Visit your skin doctor at least once a year for a complete exam in addition to your own self-exams.

The more sun exposure you have at an earlier age, the better your chances are of reaping the unfortunate results of too much ultraviolet rays. However, the more diligent you are about skin self-examination, the better your chances are of healthier skin and spotting any problems from the start.

So while it may not be the most important thing on your mind, it is important to do your own regular skin exams.

Tips on how to combat the glow of oily skin during the summer months

While wearing sunglasses to combat glare from the sun, remember to wear sunscreen on your face to combat glare from that oily glow. Just because you spend more time in the sun doesn't mean your face is tighter and drier. Sometimes not being hydrated enough and using the wrong products on your face will have opposite results.

You can end up with shiny, oily skin when you expected that sun-kissed glow.

What to put on your face

A great way to reduce the negative effects of the sun on your face is to use a suitable sunscreen with moisturizer instead of your regular moisturizer. By using your regular moisturizer and then adding sunscreen, you may be adding too much moisture.

Adding too much moisture tends to clog pores, give the appearance of oily, oily skin, and also cause acne breakouts. Before summer comes around, do some research, shop and ask for samples. Try some products to see if your skin is sensitive to them and find one that you like.

Putting a sunscreen on your face that contains moisturizer not only saves you from oily skin, it also saves you some money and a little time.

Also, see if you can give up covering your entire face with base, rather than opting for some cover-up that has a nice shiny tint.

What you put inside your body

Be sure to eat plenty of fruits and vegetables that will hydrate your skin. The fruits and vegetables that come out in the summer are generally already the most hydrating type:

* Watermelon

* Cantaloupe

* Honeydew melon

* Different types of lettuce

* Cucumbers

* Zucchini

* Blueberries, Raspberries, Grapes

Just as important as fruits and vegetables is the need for adequate hydration. Hydration can come in the form of water, plain and simple. However, if you are not a big fan, there are so many creative alternatives to just plain old water.

* Water with lemon or lime

* Homemade Iced Tea - either regular or green tea

* Good old fashioned lemonade

* Fruit smoothies with all the fresh summer fruits and vegetables

Paying attention to what you put on your face and what you put inside your body in the form of fruits, vegetables, and hydrating fluids will ensure that you don't get that oily, greasy look, and too much sunscreen off your face.

Chapter 16

The many ways that drinking water affects your skin and body

We have all heard about the benefits of drinking water, and lots of it, for weight loss and dieting. However, it is so essential for your skin, hair and body to drink water to maintain good health, especially during the summer months.

One of the biggest benefits of drinking water during the summer months is staying hydrated. Staying hydrated benefits not only your organs, but your skin as well.

The old saying that beauty is only superficial does not apply when you drink the right amount of water. Drinking the correct amount of water helps your body in many ways.

Dark circles under the eyes

Sometimes the dark circles under the eyes are really due to a lack of a good night's sleep or perhaps due to genetics. However, dark circles under the eyes are sometimes caused by lack of hydration.

Drinking more water along the way can possibly reduce those puffy dark circles. If your body needs more water, it will retain whatever it has for storage purposes. By drinking more, you can ease puffiness around the eye area.

Color, tone and texture of the skin.

Take a good look at your skin on days when it doesn't have good color, tone, and texture. Keep a journal if you like, as this will help you see firsthand the benefits of drinking extra water in the summer.

When you spend time in the hot summer sun, you will notice that your skin will look drier, no matter what you do or how many cosmetics you put on your face. The best moisturizer is water.

Acne

Isn't it better to treat your skin properly from the start than to buy many expensive acne treatments, which could only end up drying your skin over time? By drinking additional water in summer, it provides a natural cleanser for your skin and pores. The water serves as a cleanser and exfoliant and to prevent acne.

Dryness and peeling

If you are like any other person, you have had the experience of staying in the sun too long and burning yourself, especially in the facial areas. By drinking additional water, it provides a natural barrier for the skin to stay hydrated and moist. Dryness and exfoliation will heal much faster the more water you absorb.

Since the body is made up of over 70% water, it stands to reason that it needs water to survive and thrive, especially in the summer.

Chapter 17

Skincare Tips for Women of Color

When people think of someone who is beautiful, it is often based on both inner beauty and outer beauty. Both are under your control to change. You really need to have both to look your best. Here are some tips to start your own personal beauty adventure.

For a convenient container to carry some of your favorite moisturizer, fill a small bottle or an empty lip gloss container. This perfectly portable container can be kept in your purse, car, travel bag or even in your desk drawer at work. When your skin begins to dry, apply a drop of moisturizer.

Invest the extra money in a set of quality makeup brushes. Remember, these tools will touch your face every day. If you spend more on these brushes, you can get a set that will last for years. You should also pick up a bottle of brush cleaner, which should be used regularly, at least twice a week. This eliminates dust and bacteria.

Put petroleum jelly on your eyebrows before going to sleep. This will make your eyebrows look better and brighter. Avoid getting petroleum jelly anywhere else on the face because it can cause unwanted acne breakouts.

If you have striking brown eyes, you can play them by adding eyeshadow, liner, and mascara in colors that are especially flattering for your eye color. Look for rich, matte shades in shades of green, copper, and blue. These colors add depth and intensity to the color of your eyes, especially when covered with a few layers of navy blue mascara.

To play green or hazel eyes and create a candlelight effect, choose eye colors that highlight the shades of gold and green in your irises. If you have green or hazel eyes, use colors that are light brown, lavender, and other shades of purple.

Baking soda can enhance the shine of your hair! Just put a little baking soda in the shampoo you will be using. Wash your hair as usual. This eliminates product build-up and leaves your hair shiny and clean.

To make your feet look beautiful, especially during the warmer, drier summer months, try applying petroleum jelly every day. It will keep them smooth and soft. Then get yourself a pedicure and a whole new pair of daring sandals, and you'll have the best feet of the season.

Avoid licking your lips. When you constantly lick your lips, instead of getting wet, they actually dry out. Try carrying a lip balm or gloss in your pocket or purse, and put it on whenever you feel like licking a little. You will soon find your lips in perfect condition.

Place the mirror under your face when you put on eye shadow. Avoid pulling or pressing on the eyelids. Be sure to look down, which will help you get the right app the first time. Apply your shadow carefully, and you won't need to stretch the lid.

Keep the top of your head a top priority when styling your hair. This area is more difficult to design and if you are tired once you get close to that area it can ruin your whole look.

To avoid breakouts and maintain pure makeup colors, you should wash your makeup brushes frequently. Use a mild soap and warm water to rinse until the water runs clear. Rinse applicators well, then allow to dry with a clean hand towel. This helps prevent makeup from building up. It also kills bacteria that can damage your skin and cause acne.

You learned from the beginning of this article that it is important to have both inner beauty and outer beauty to be considered truly beautiful. It may look pretty at first, although if you have a bad personality, its beauty will disappear very quickly. Follow the advice this article has given you to take your beauty to the next level.

Chapter 18

Bonus: Beauty is not easier than this

You don't have to be incredibly strict with beauty to fully enjoy it. Not at all! You can apply whatever you want, as it can also be a relaxing activity. If you have no idea how to get started, try looking at the tips below. They can give you some useful advice.

No matter how your skin looks and feels, it is important to wash your face at least once a day. Regardless of your personal beauty regimen, get in the habit of always removing all of your makeup completely before cleaning your face. If you don't properly clean your face, it can cause clogged pores and often acne.

The color of your hair should influence which cosmetic colors suit you best. For example, if you are a brunette, you can use a dark mahogany eyeshadow as a multitasking tool. In a pinch, it can be used to fill in scattered eyebrows, align the upper lash line, and even cover the gray roots in the hairline.

Before spending the night, wash off your makeup to save your skin. Gently rub your face with a warm washcloth. Clean your face with other products thereafter. If you don't remove your makeup properly, your pores may become clogged and acne may appear.

Replace aloe gel with expensive moisturizers, witch hazel with expensive toners, and pure castile soap with a clean cloth for high-priced cleaners. When you use organic and natural elements, your skin will instantly light up. If you need even more moisture, add a little vitamin E. If medicinal tonics are required, you can always add a little tea tree oil.

To improve your lip color application, always apply the lip balm first. The lip balm will leave your lips soft and hydrated, and will allow your lip color to continue smoothly. Try using a basic, undyed lip balm to avoid affecting the color of the lipstick or the lip gloss you're wearing.

Beauty tip for tired eyes! The eye gel will help reduce the appearance of puffy or tired eyes. Keep this in the fridge and use it for an extra boost if you're really tired. You can feel very tired without having to show it on your face. Just be sure to use the gel on a clean face.

Put your vegetables on your skin. Vegetables have many health benefits when you eat them, and several more when used as a beauty treatment. Try cold cucumbers or sliced potatoes on your eyes to relieve puffiness and redness. Use the remaining water from boiling cabbage, broccoli, or kale for a healthy skin tonic.

Choose your eyeshadow based on your eye color so your eye makeup really stands out. If your eyes are blue, brown tones are the most flattering. For brown eyes, try purple shades like lavender or plum. If your eyes are green, the shades of gold are very flattering, as are many shades of the brown family.

A little beauty tip from the main makeup artists to look rested even when it is not to avoid accumulating in the base. Try using a tinted moisturizer instead, and then apply a beige eyeliner, this will counteract the redness around the eyes and make you look refreshed and ready for the day.

One way to avoid wrinkling eyeshadow, as much oil as possible should be removed from the eyelids. It's easy to do using a pressed powder or eyeshadow base before applying color. These help absorb any oil on the eyelids and prevent the eyeshadow from wrinkling.

Look, beauty is more than precision based. If not, only professionals could buy and use the products. You should feel a little better and ready to start and practice in order to use your new knowledge.

Choosing the right makeup for your face

The world of beauty is very vast and exciting. There are many ways that one can earn, and then use the knowledge in this field to help them feel more secure and attractive. It depends entirely on the individual. With that said, no matter what your beauty skills are, here are some tips you'll find extremely helpful.

New products called mattifying lotions are perfect for any makeup kit because they can be applied to any part of the face that seems slippery from excess oils. These lotions often have a creamy or thick gel consistency and can be applied without a mirror; it also provides a soft foundation on which makeup can be applied.

You can easily exfoliate your face lightly during your daily bath or shower using a soft, knotty towel or wash cloth. This is especially effective if the water is warm, not hot, and only if you are using the cloth for the first time. Never use the same cloth two days in a row as bacteria can build up overnight.

Brighten up your eyes with this natural look: apply a clear, neutral colored eyeshadow all over your upper eyelid. Look for sand, khaki, beige, or beige colors. This will neutralize any redness on your eyelids, which can make you look older and tired. Add drama by smearing a darker shade on the tops only in the crease.

Sometimes skin blemishes like pimples can detract from our beauty at the most inopportune times. Use a little toothpaste to combat any stains that appear on your skin. Let the toothpaste dry for about 10 minutes. This should dramatically reduce the appearance of the grain.

Use a deep conditioner at least once a week for extra smooth and healthy hair. Choose a day of the week to bathe and read a magazine or listen to music while the deep conditioner penetrates your hair before rinsing it off. Many lines of hair products include a matching deep conditioner.

You don't need to spend a lot of money on a stylish deep conditioning mask. There are many recipes you can make at home that include nutrient-dense foods that are great for your hair. An excellent one includes strawberry puree and enough mayonnaise to make a spread. Leave it on your wet hair for 10 minutes and rinse.

Make your skin more beautiful by eating fruit. If you have a sweet tooth and you fill it with sugar, you can quickly see it on your skin. You can feed your sweet tooth and your skin by eating sweet fruit instead of something sugary. When you do this, your skin will not be the sole beneficiary.

Apply a lotion or cream that contains sunscreen every day. You have to live your whole life with the same skin and it is worth investing to protect it. You should start each day with a layer of sunscreen before you even think about going out. Your skin will thank you.

Boar bristle brushes can be helpful in counteracting frizzy hair. Many people suffer from frizzy hair. Using a boar bristle brush on dry hair can help you fight frizz. While gently brushing your hair, make sure the blow dryer is pointing down.

Beauty is a fascinating and exciting world that is only limited by the reach of a person's imagination. There are infinite possibilities, products, combinations and techniques. Start experimenting to find something new for yourself or to learn something new that you can improve for your own use. Get inspired with these tips!

Ideas that will make you look like a star

There are plenty of chic products promoted by glamorous Hollywood models and actresses, but don't give in to this high pressure! Your lips are thin, your eyes are too far apart, and your nose looks weird. That's not the truth! There is a lot of information available that will help you look better and stay positive. Read on for some great tips to make you look your best!

Beautiful Skin

Lightly spray your face with a hydrating mist to make your makeup last longer. The mist will help you set up your makeup, keep it fresh, and give you that freshly made-up makeup look for hours. This is great for keeping your makeup in place during those long days at work or late nights out with friends.

You can prevent sun damage to your skin by using a good sunscreen. When examining the many sunscreen options, it makes sense to opt for ones that contain organic or healthy ingredients and antioxidants. These healthy ingredients protect and nourish the skin, keeping it young and supple.

Before applying a fake tan, be sure to remove unwanted hair at least 24 hours before doing so. You can shave or shave, but be sure to do it more than a day later. This will help ensure that the tan is pleasant, even and smooth.

Wear gloves when applying suntan lotions and keep a towel close to you. This will help you if you make a mess and keep your palms from turning orange or tan. You should also make sure to pull your hair back so that your tan is applied evenly.

Wash your face before going to sleep. This will remove all the impurities and dirt from the day. Use a make-up remover first, to remove makeup, then use a face wash. If you don't clean your face before bed, your pores can become clogged and cause pimples or blemishes.

Always have moisturizer with you if you want your skin to be perfect. This is especially important during winter. Cold weather can crack and damage your skin. Keeping the skin constantly moisturized can prevent dryness and any breakage or cracking.

If you want to restore the shine of your hair, you can use baking soda! Use a little baking soda mixed with your shampoo before washing. Wash your hair as usual. This brings shine to your hair.

To help your liner last all day, apply a thin layer of eyeshadow in a matching color over the top. Most eyeliners tend to fade or run throughout the day. This is particularly true for oil-based eye pencils. You can eliminate this problem by brushing a matching eyeshadow layer directly over the top of the liner with a thin makeup brush. This helps configure it to stay in place all day.

If you want to have good skin, naturally drink plenty of water. Water naturally helps cleanse your body of toxins, and this action gives you beautiful, clear skin throughout the day.

Extend your base by adding a moisturizer to the bottle. This also gives you a healthy glow against a "cakey" appearance and adds SPF to your skin.

Apply eyeshadow to seal the liner. When you are putting on your eyes, apply your eyeliner before your eyeshadow. Then when you apply the shadow, lightly moisten a cotton swab and add a bit of eyeshadow. Smooth this over the siding and you will see it last much longer.

Finding what works best for you can be a little difficult since the world is full of supermodels and ridiculously expensive products. Hopefully, you've learned some solid advice on how to make yourself feel and look more beautiful! Don't be afraid to experiment and enjoy your new look with greater confidence.

Ideas to find your own beauty and style

Looking beautiful is something that can make any woman feel good about herself. It is important to take the time to pamper yourself and spend some time on your beauty routine. This article will give you a lot of advice on how to improve the beauty that you naturally have every day.

Keep your eye gel in your refrigerator. This can help soothe puffy eyes or dark circles around the eyes. Cool eye gel can really make your eyes look cool after a long night. Just apply it as you normally would to see immediate, all-day results.

Soften the corners of your face with a soft coral or creamy pink blush. Place the blush on the cheekbones and then, with your fingers, spread it outward toward the temples.

If your face is slightly elongated, you can make the effect appear less severe by simply using a little well-placed cream blush. Go for a dark rose or brick tone, then use your fingertips to apply the color only to the apples of your cheeks; do not extend the color beyond this point, as it can make your face appear even narrower.

Curl your lashes with an eyelash curler before putting on your mask. This will make them look longer and will make your eyes look alert and bright. Start by squeezing the curling iron at the bottom of the lashes and holding it for a short time. Once you have done that, move your lashes and repeat the squeeze motion. Doing this adds a natural look to the curl you're giving your lashes.

When you get up in the morning, you must pamper yourself. The best way to start your day on the right foot is to take time to brush your hair, wash your face, and brush your teeth. Don't neglect your own needs if you want to stay beautiful.

If the thought of applying false lash strips gives you cold feet, consider individual lashes instead. These are considerably easier to apply and require only a small amount of eyelash glue, compared to the amount used for full lashes. Individual lashes, when placed in the outer corner of the eyes, produce a much more natural effect.

Don't forget that your hands must also be pampered. Hands are often overlooked in beauty treatments. So it is said, if you want to know someone's age, check their hands. In addition to daily lotion or cream treatment, you should exfoliate your hands once a week.

If you have dry skin, or older looking skin, you should exfoliate weekly. You should also do this if you are applying some form of tanning lotion. You must exfoliate first to get the most out of the tanning lotion you are using.

Turn up your hair color. If you have dyed your hair and the results are not as dramatic as you would like, you can fix this by adding a box of hair coloring to your shampoo. Roll it into your hair and let it sit for 5 minutes, then rinse it off.

To open pores and remove blemishes, steam is a wonderful option. Place your face on a bowl of steaming hot water with a dry towel placed over your head. Do this as long as you are careful not to burn yourself. When you've had enough, splash your face with cold water to close your pores and make your skin firmer.

Beautiful Skin

There have been many beauty tips in this article. Have fun and have a girls night out where you and your friends can try many of these tips. Making yourself a little more beautiful should always be fun, and it will always have a good result.

Solid advice when trying to make yourself look good

Beauty lies within, but improving the exterior never hurts! Most people want to emphasize its natural characteristics. Learn how to shine using the tips in this article.

Sunscreen keeps your skin flawless. When examining the many sunscreen options, it makes sense to opt for ones that contain organic or healthy ingredients and antioxidants. You can keep your skin younger and firmer with the right rich protective ingredients.

If you only have the time and money for a single beauty product, consider spending it on a flattering cheek color. A cream-based blush is easily applied using only your fingertips and can be thrown into your bag and applied quickly and with little or no effort. This is an item you shouldn't be afraid to spend a little more on.

Use a warm toner or moisturizer for the skin to refresh and add color to dull skin. Get a natural shine by using a sponge to apply bronzer to the cheekbones and brow bones. To prevent it from looking shiny, just apply the moisturizer to the apple of your cheeks and under the eyebrows.

Use a misting spray to set makeup. Once you have finished putting on your makeup, spray lightly with a spray bottle. This will set up your makeup, keeping it in place longer before requiring you to touch it up. This is perfect for long night outings or events like weddings.

If you want to stay beautiful, keep your skin healthy and feel good, drink plenty of water! 5-8 glasses of water a day is great, and even more is always good if you can handle it. Drinking lots of water helps with bad or dry skin and many other ailments.

Keep your makeup light and simple. If you put on too much makeup you can stress your skin and make you look older than you are. The best beauty is often the least complicated. Maintain your routine with a quality moisturizer, followed by lip gloss and a good mascara.

For an inexpensive spa facial, just lean into a bowl of hot, steaming water! Cover or wrap your hair, fill any container with very hot water, and let the steam open and clear your pores! It is soothing and stimulating and very profitable. Follow up with cold water to tighten and refresh pores, then add moisturizer!

To get even more out of your favorite eye gel, keep it in the fridge! The ingredients in the eye gel work hard to restore and protect the delicate skin around the eyes and keeping it cool improves the refresh factor tenfold! The cold will also work right away to reduce that horrible swelling!

If you wear your hair in a ponytail frequently, move the ponytail position from time to time to avoid breaking your hair. Constant stress and friction on the same part of the hair shaft can weaken the hair, but placing the rubber or elastic band in different positions prevents the same spots from being rubbed over and over again.

If you suffer from chronic, dry skin, you may want to see a dermatologist and get a microdermabrasion facial peel. Microdermabrasions can improve skin function and appearance in no time. A treatment will help your skin feel softer and improve the elasticity of your skin. Although one treatment helps, for the best results you should schedule at least 6 treatments.

So if you want to improve the exterior that's understandable, most people do! Minimizing your failures and highlighting your assets is the best plan. The advice in this article is sure to help you do both. These tips can help you be beautiful on the outside and inside.

The best beauty tip everyone should know

Finding valuable tips, advice and information on what to include in your daily beauty regimen is essential to get the look you are looking for. Knowing the best application and preparation methods will make it much easier for you to get beautiful skin, as well as the glow of your overall self that everyone wants to have.

The scientific definition of beauty is symmetry. Try to maintain your symmetry when fighting for beauty. Regardless of whether you're trimming your beard or putting on makeup, you need to make sure the left and right sides are symmetrical (mirror images).

Apply a light moisturizer before applying a fake tan on your skin. A fake tan will build up on dry skin spots. You need to make sure you pay attention to your feet, elbows, knees, and around your wrists. Apply lotion to these areas before applying a fake bronzer.

These procedures can leave hair follicles open, and tanning may cause some skin problems. You can experience significant irritation if you choose to tan. Do not use fragrance-free products after waxing; they will also cause irritation.

Do you want clear, clean and healthy skin? Exfoliation is essential! Exfoliate your skin regularly to remove all the trash, chemicals, and dirt you are exposed to every day. The internet has many great recipes for scrubs that cleanse your skin naturally and without costing you an arm and a leg - check it out!

Always take off your makeup before bed. If you sleep with makeup on, your chances of acne and blackheads increase. Makeup can trap dirt and oil on the face. Clean and tone your face every night. Don't forget to add moisturizer when you're done cleaning.

Use bright eyeshadows in your beauty routine. Because shiny particles in makeup reflect light, these shades can create the illusion of bigger, brighter eyes. Look for spotted shades that are close to your skin color. Don't hesitate to experiment with different techniques and colors.

To cleanse your skin without depriving it of its natural oils, use a cream cleanser. A cream cleanser will help retain healthy skin oils on your face and will also leave your face hydrated and shiny. Using this type of cleaner will delay the development of fine lines and wrinkles.

If you're like many who have trouble keeping your liner where it's supposed to be, try applying your eyeshadow to the top of the liner with a damp cotton ball. It will help set up the siding and hold it in place longer than you would otherwise.

Keep in mind what certain colors and patterns look like as your body changes over time. Just as styles can change over time, so can your hair color and skin tones. Therefore, colors that did not complement it in the past can complement it now. Also, the opposite may be true. The colors you found fantastic may not look great on you now. Find out which ones make you look good and stay away from the ones that don't.

To help you pluck your eyebrows, you should hold the tweezers upright against the side of your nose. Then you move the clamps along your eyebrows, and you will easily see where your arch should start and stop. This will ensure that you stick with the natural shape of your eyebrows.

Hopefully, you have found the information provided to you to be quite informative and useful. Knowing these tips can be the first step to get the results you are looking for. Apply these tips to your beauty regimen and the healthy skin you are looking for will surely come to you.

Chapter 19

Conclusion

As featured, there are many ways to achieve and maintain a beautiful skin. All you need to consider is to make some efforts to change your habits. Eating nutritious foods like those mentioned above is perhaps one of the most necessary movements to consider if you want beautiful skin. Just think clean and green and have beautiful skin.

The dermatologist is the professional who knows best and can guide the most appropriate measures for skin care in each individual, using the most effective and reliable diagnostic methods.

If you liked this book I invite you to leave me a Review to continue writing this type of content, it helps a lot and I will be very grateful.

See you soon in the next book!!!

Best Regards,,

Francisco V. Giulepp